The Virgin Diet Supreme

Fast Weight Loss Logic

By Cathy Wilson

Copyright © 2014

Income Disclaimer

This book contains business strategies, marketing methods and other business advice that, regardless of my own results and experience, may not produce the same results (or any results) for you. I make absolutely no guarantee, expressed or implied, that by following the advice below you will make any money or improve current profits, as there are several factors and variables that come into play regarding any given business.

Primarily, results will depend on the nature of the product or business model, the conditions of the marketplace, the experience of the individual, and situations and elements that are beyond your control.

As with any business endeavor, you assume all risk related to investment and money based on your own discretion and at your own potential expense.

Liability Disclaimer

By reading this book, you assume all risks associated with using the advice given below, with a full understanding that you, solely, are responsible for anything that may occur as a result of putting this information into action in any way, and regardless of your interpretation of the advice.

You further agree that our company cannot be held responsible in any way for the success or failure of your business as a result of the information presented in this book. It is your responsibility to conduct your own due diligence regarding the safe and successful operation of your business if you intend to apply any of our information in any way to your business operations.

Terms of Use

You are given a non-transferable, "personal use" license to this book. You cannot distribute it or share it with other individuals.

Also, there are no resale rights or private label rights granted when purchasing this book. In other words, it's for your own personal use only.

The Virgin Diet Supreme

Fast Weight Loss Logic

By Cathy Wilson

Table of Contents

Overview of Virgin Diet

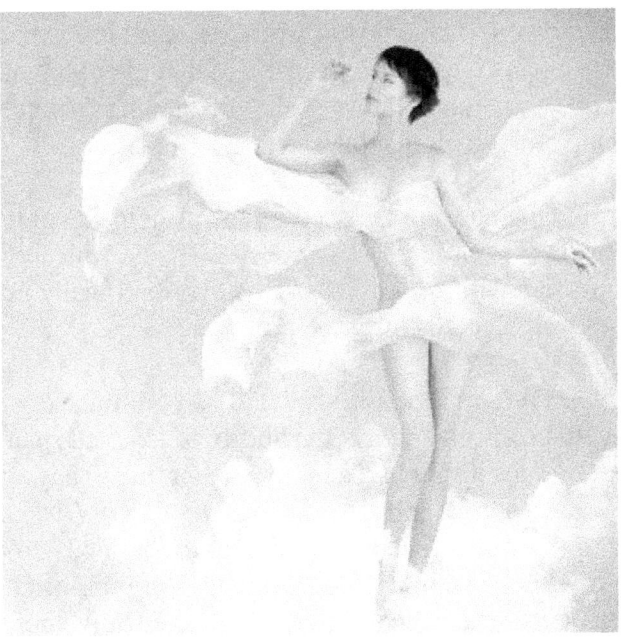

My perception is to think outside the box when it comes to dieting. Opening your mind see the positives and negatives, focusing on the take action information to sharpen your personal health and wellness decisions.

If you learn just one positive change that betters you from my masterpiece, then I'm one happy lady!

FOCUS – Making positive health changes that are sustainable and even enjoyable for YOU!

Fact is, there isn't any one diet, or way of eating, that's perfect for everyone. There's always something you could be doing differently or better, to lower the risk of disease, drop a few pounds more, or flip your frown upside down faster.

If you've got knowledge and willpower, there IS a way. These are the tools of change.

With the Virgin Diet concept, there really is a whole lot of positive. I'm going to fill you up with quality introductory facts, and it's up to you to take this information, the stuff that makes sense to you, and apply it to your life. You never know unless you try, and your job is figuring out what health changes sends fat packing and which just interfere.

The Virgin Diet concept is based on the principal people have food intolerances or allergies to specific foods, which ultimately can interfere with weight loss. This is scientifically proven, so put your argue cards away please!

When these conflict foods are isolated and eliminated, your body regains control, and has the ability to lose fat, steer off disease, and stay strong and healthy. All in theory anyway. *JJ Virgin* does a great job introducing *The Virgin Diet* eating strategy to the world. She does claim up to 7 pounds dropped in a week, which is a little steep. At least 7 pounds of fat is, simply because when according to *Dietician* Daily, there's a whopping 3,500 calories in just one pound! Which means you'd have to 24,500 less calories in that week, and or expend that much extra energy on top of the calories it takes to sustain your weight, with a combination of increased exercise, and major calorie slashing.

Regardless, experts agree that's extreme for most, and truly unhealthy, considering the average size healthy woman consumes 2,000 - 2,500 calories per day.

According to WebMD, it's safe to lose 2-3 pounds per week, with healthy eating, and plenty of exercise. My Virgin Diet Supreme, shows you how to safely lose weight at a steady pace and sustain your weight loss. The key to fat blasting success!

Slow, steady, and smart healthy adjustments wins the race in sustained weight loss. I've added to The Virgin Diet concept, including more emphasis on factors outside of eating, where the backup dancing need more attention. Cuz I don't care who you are, losing weight the right way and keeping it off, isn't happening without attention to realities like, improved lifestyle, affective exercise, and better life perspective.

Focusing to make positive health and wellness change outside the food factor, is only going to bump you closer to your weight loss goals sooner.

Is your glass half full or half empty?
One early issue worth your attention, is that food intolerance is something you can develop somewhere in utero, or any time throughout life. Which makes it incredibly difficult to gage what foods are mucking up your system, and to what degree. Just something to keep in mind while you read through The Virgin Diet Supreme.

Essentially what happens with this eating concept is, the first week you vamoose these potentially allergenic foods from your menu. After this first cycle is complete, you start reintroducing these foods singularly, to figure out which ones are interfering with your bodily system function, and which are innocent of ruckus.

These are the seven foods you aren't allowed to eat for the first week, why, and alternatives:
* **Dairy** - Milk is very high in lactose, a sugar that may cause insulin resistance over time, triggering blood sugar issues found in people with diabetes. Experts also agree dairy can trigger skin problems, and milk isn't the only food that helps maintain growth and strong bones. Calcium is also found in leafy green veggies, seeds and nuts, minus the negative reac-

11

tion in most cases. So you needn't fret about not getting your protein, calcium and essential vitamins!

Ideas: Unsweetened almond of coconut milk instead of cow milk, coconut milk yogurt instead of cow milk yogurt, and sugar-free coconut milk ice cream instead of the regular stuff.

* Eggs - Up to 65% of people have some sort of egg intolerance. Eggs are also very high in pro-inflammatory arachidonic acid.

Ideas: Have a protein smoothie instead of an egg omelet, eat free-range eggs if you must on occasion.

* Gluten -This triggers a protein release called zonulin, which loosens up your small intestine, allowing more food particles to slip through and cause inflammation and negative immune response.

Ideas: Use rice or romaine wraps instead of wheat, spaghetti squash instead of pasta, and quinoa in place of couscous.

* Soy - Most is modified genetically and loaded with harmful pesticides, and other toxins your body absorbs and can't digest. Soy damages the gut, and often unknowingly interferes with your thyroid function.

Ideas: Almond or coconut milk instead of soymilk, sugar-free coconut milk ice cream instead of soy ice cream, and sometimes fermented soy works, like miso.

* Sugar/Sweeteners - Of course sugar triggers lots of problems, but artificial sweeteners are worse, triggering insulin response which interferes with weight loss and causes weight gain.

Ideas: Skip the sugar and sweeteners and try monk fruit, Stevia or erythritol, and enjoy natural sweeteners like vanilla and pure cinnamon.

* **Peanuts** - They are often associated with mold and a trouble-some fungus called aflatoxin. They're also high in fructose corn syrup and Trans fats. A deadly synthetic fat that poisons your body.
Ideas: Nuts/seeds and almonds instead of peanuts, and almond butter instead of peanut butter works.

* **Corn** - It has high sugar, often modified genetically, and triggers inflammation.
Ideas: Have quinoa or legumes instead of corn, raw veggies work instead of the ever popular popcorn.

This diet plan works with 3 cycles of 7 days.
* **First Cycle** - Remove top hi-fi food choices - up to seven pounds can be lost

* **Second Cycle** - Re-introduce one of the most reactive foods to your body: eggs, dairy, soy, and gluten

* **Third Cycle** - Here you will devise a plan including exercise, with the information you've gained from the previous two cycles. The goal is to create new life habits that are going to better your health and wellness long-term. Once each year you will eliminate those 7 highly allergenic foods to cleanse your system.
Pretty straight forward and makes sense.

My Thoughts . . .
The Virgin Diet works by troubleshooting the foods you are currently eating that may be interfering with your good health. Causing you to feel lethargic, gain weight, get moody, easily irritated, and trigger avoidable symptoms of disease and illness, that are going to stress you and negatively interfere with daily function.

By getting to the root of your health issues and removing them, you will have an opening to create an eating strategy that accommodates your personal preferences and tolerances, according to your body and mind.

You are unique, and over time your system may decide it doesn't think too kindly towards specific foods, particular dairy and wheat products, which may interfere with the running of your system.

There often is no rhyme or reason for this, it just is.
The Virgin Diet eliminates foods most likely to cause issue with your body, then slowly re-introduces them back into your daily diet, so you can decide if you're booting them out or not.

After which, you can recreate an eating plan that will give you all the essential vitamins and minerals your body requires to be strong and healthy, without supporting stress.. Taking a good supplement, especially during this first week, is also a smart move.

This eating tactic often uncovers solutions to the frustrations people have losing weight, why energy levels are down, and how come specific foods irritate their internal systems as a whole. The least that will happen, is you're going to gain peace of mind knowing what foods work for your body best.

Cycles in Action

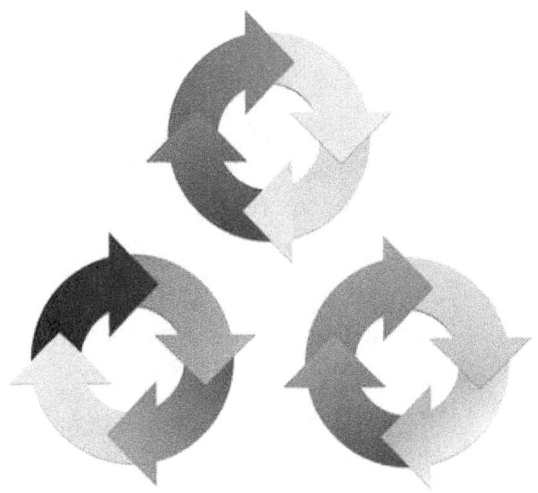

It's important we dig beneath the surface to understand how these three cycles work, what they include, and how to take action with your newfound knowledge. You can be the sharpest matchstick in the box, but if you don't know **how** to implement, you're never getting past glowing embers.

First Cycle to Transform

By shocking your system through the elimination of numerous well-used foods, you're likely going to drop a significant amount of weight off the top. Experts agree, this fast weight loss is a positive, because studies show that

healthy fast weight loss has a greater chance of staying off, when compared to those pesky pounds that seem to take forever to disappear.

Again, the seven hi-fi foods you're eliminating are:
* Corn
* Sugar/sweetener
* Gluten
* Dairy
* Soy
* Peanuts
* Eggs

KEY FACTOR - If you cheat here, then you aren't going to get the results you need and deserve. You *MUST* eliminate all of these foods, and commit to steering completely clear of them for 7 days. If you even have a "taste" of any one of them,

you've gotta go back to the drawing board, if you want a fair shot reaching your health and wellness goals with The Virgin Diet.

Do I make myself crystal clear?

The Purpose?

Gives your body a chance to recover from the potential stresses of these foods. Of course you're speculating, but the only way to figure out without a doubt, what foods are interfering with your great health and lack of fat loss, is to get rid of them **all** for 7 days!

You can expect to "feel" all sorts of annoying aches and pains diminishing during this first cycle, including:
* Inflammation issues
* Joint pain and headaches
* Bloating and gas
* Extreme tiredness
* Hazy thinking fog
* Annoying creaks and cracks

Research studies show, it's your immune complexes that are triggering many of these symptoms. So if you are eating even a few of these "forbidden" foods, you're triggering the release of IgG antibodies, and manifesting your health issues.

Eventually you'll shift laterally, and replace these hi-fi foods.

You will consume "the right" foods, the ones that will help your body gain strength, increase immunity, level blood sugars, decrease swelling and inflammation in general, better digestion, and help you drop fat.

Nourishment to flush these 7 "trigger-some" foods from your diet - The Process:
First - Begin each morning with what's called a Virgin Shake.
- Berries
- Flax seed
- Coconut milk (unsweetened)
- Rice/pea protein
This shake is very tasty and filling, gives you energy, and leaves you feeling happy, happy, happy.

Second - Each meal enables you to customize your eating, and includes:
- Lean protein - free range beef/poultry, pea/rice protein and wild fish are better choices
- Lots of leafy vegetables
- High-fiber complex carbohydrates - quinoa, lentils and legumes, and sweet potato

Health Alert - Quinoa is also a complete protein that's plant based, and excellent for your diet!
- Good fats used sparingly - olive oil, coconut oil/milk, seeds, nuts, and avocado

Health Alert - Unsaturated fats like olive oil and sunflower oil, are labeled "good fats." They tend to be liquid at room temperature, and help to give your body the 25-30% fat it needs to thrive. However, coconut oil is considered a saturated fat, even though it provides countless health benefits proven scientifically: From clearing up skin conditions, to strengthening your natural resistance to disease and illness. Coconut oil is technically classified as a saturated fat, but is the exception to the rule in moderation.

Essentially, you're looking to replace one or two meals each day with your "Virgin Shake," to help heal your digestive system.

I'm sure you've heard, people seem to lose a significant amounts of weight during this initial phase, by eliminating these seven hi-fi foods from their diet. Shocking the system, and naturally eliminating a whole whack of fat calories you'd otherwise be eating.

Think of this as a bonus for your efforts. Understanding if you don't continue on track with the program, you're selling yourself short on the benefits of your new learned eating strategy.

Second Cycle to Customize
Congrats! You have cleansed out your system and will feel energized and alive. It's time to shift into second gear.

This is where the personalization or custom design comes into play. This is where you find out what foods are welcome, and which aren't for your body. You are unique, as are your internal system functions, preferences, tolerances, and limitations. In the second cycle, you're going to re-introduce a single hi-fi food at a time; soy, gluten, eggs, and dairy.

The idea is to try one of these 7 foods for 4 days, and avoid it for 3. If you don't experience any negative reactions, then your system is fine with it. Of course if you react, then it's best to steer clear.

* My math isn't THAT bad. The three other hi-fi foods - sugars/sweeteners, peanuts and corn - should be permanently removed or ate very sparingly.

Most people eat all these elimination foods, thinking they are perfectly healthy, and many of them are. The flip side is, they often unknowingly interfere with your natural body systems for a multitude of reasons. By taking the time to troubleshoot your eating with the "Virgin Diet" strategies, you're going to help your body run smooth and efficiently, ultimately optimizing your health.

Your good health and well-being's worth a few months of non-invasive investigation in my expert opinion.

Third Cycle to Sustain

Here, you're going to gain knowledge in the "how to" department. The theory is, if you don't know how to use the strategies you've learned to keep the weight off for good, then you've just got another pipe dream. A short-term fad diet toiling with your emotions. Delivering unbelievable hope and happiness one minute, and slapping you in the face with weight gain reality the next.

The Virgin Diet was created to set you up for long-term weight loss success, and toss in the bonus of preventative measures for various diseases, including breast cancer. It teaches sensible and reasonable eating tactics, that your brain will love, and we all know it's your noggin that's driving your boat, most of the time anyway.

The majority of diets on the market, show you quick and drastic ways to drop flubber, but fail to address anything after you reach the finish line.

NEWSFLASH! There shouldn't be a finish line with any effective eating strategy. The mindset you create with The Virgin Diet, is to make smart food choices that are sustainable forever. In time you'll transform these new decisions into habit, and that thought's gotta make you smile!

It's safe to say, optimal health and wellness, including maintain a healthy weight, has numerous factors that come into play. Exercise and a positive lifestyle in general will definitely reflect your ability to use The Virgin Diet as a lifelong platform, to continuously raise your health upwards towards bigger and better.

The third cycle is where you start implementing regular exercise. Although this isn't a focus, it's important to start slow and work your way up. Cardiovascular exercise intertwined with weight training and strength training, is only going to help you internal systems work more effectively, blasting fat, and increasing your energy levels, leaving you feeling, thinking, and looking, fantabulous!

At this point, it's also critical once a year to repeat the first cycle. Every day your body is changing, and you could potentially develop a new resistance to a food you had no trouble with the previous year. For this reason it's important to take the time to check in each year and repeat the first cycle, because you're worth it.

My Thoughts . . .
Knowing what to expect, and how to execute each phase of a diet plan prior to experiencing it, is important. This diet makes sense. It's a great way to gather the information you need, to pinpoint foods you tolerate, and ones you don't.

Think long term here, because that's what The Virgin Diet is all about. Healthy and sustainable eating that is enjoyable, and will stand the test of time, versatile and diverse, which are very important in making sure you stick with this healthy eating strategy for life.

The Culprit Explained - Food Intolerance

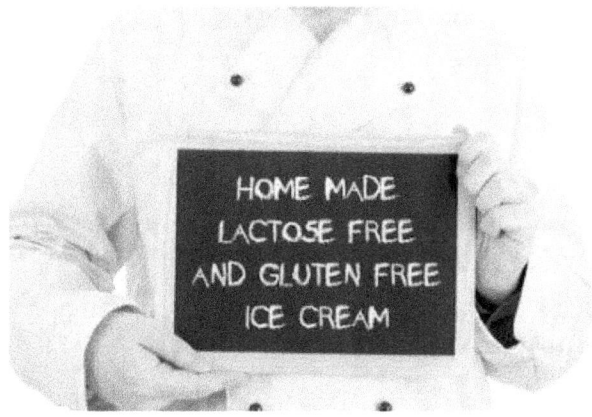

Weight loss resistance is often overlooked when determining why someone isn't losing weight, when they're seemingly doing all the "right" things to drop blubber. The Virgin Diet places this notion center stage, and explores what foods may be wreaking havoc with your weight loss efforts.

Food intolerance is also coined non-allergenic food hypersensitivity, used for numerous physiological reactions linked to a specific type of food. Before getting too far ahead, it's important you understand the difference between "food intolerance" and "food allergy."

Food Allergy Symptoms:
* Sudden and explosive
* May be life-threatening
* Occurs whenever you eat a specific food

23

* Very sensitive - just smelling the food may trigger

Food Intolerance Symptoms
* Amount of food eaten may reflect severity of symptoms
* Happens slowly
* May only surface if food is eaten often
* Not life-threatening

Here Are Some Shared Symptoms
* Stomach upset
* Gas
* Diarrhea
* Cramps
* Vomiting

The Differences from Food Intolerance
With intolerance, your stomach lining is bothered and this in-terferes with digestion.
- Tummy upset, cramps, bloating
- Gas, heartburn
- Headaches, migraines, TMJ
- Nervousness, anxiety, moodiness

With an allergy, your immune system naturally attacks food because it registers it as harmful to your system. This causes issue with your whole stomach, and not just your tummy.

- Trouble breathing
- Skin breakout - rash, hives
- Trouble swallowing
- Blood pressure drop
- Life threatening

Lactose intolerance is the most common of food intolerances. Essentially, where your system can't break down the sugar found in milk, which is lactose. More recently, intolerances to food additives has come to surface, particularly the sulphites added to foods. This can trigger acute asthma attacks.

Why Food Intolerances?
Food intolerances seem to be on the rise, which makes sense when you stop and think about it. All the natural and man-made toxins and poisons we breathe, eat and surround our-selves with, makes some sort of negative reaction inevitable. If you are loading yourself up with Trans fat soaked processed foods, and think your body is getting all the nutritious vitamins and minerals it requires to deter disease, and keep you strong and healthy for life, you're kidding yourself. All these "non-food" chemicals and preservatives that get into our system have no place to go.

This will eventually interfere with the normal intricately bal-anced systems in your body, and there WILL be some sort of consequence. A signal of your body desperately trying to tell you to "get natural" with your eating to start, comes in the form of food intolerance. It's a gentle signal that your internal mech-anisms aren't feeling too great, and you need to figure out why. Just like you heading to the dentist when you've got a tooth in-fection, and it feels like a freakin truck ran over your face.

The Virgin Diet is the best place to start.
Life is crazy busy for most, and one thing the majority of us lose is the ability to connect with our body, to actually listen. We train our body to crave junk food when hungry, by habitu-ally grabbing a candy bar to tie us over until dinner, instead of a healthy banana, or exotic starfruit. Or starving ourselves till lunch, cuz we think it's a fantastico way to lose a few pounds. Having trained your mind to believe fictitiously true hunger pains are a red flag to not eat, because it means we must be burning fat. Totally crack-head messed up.

25

Unfortunately none of the above is true, and this until we re-learn what our body wants and needs, and provide the essential vitamins and minerals it needs, along with regular exercise, we are always going to be dealing with *preventable* health issues.

FACT - Food intolerances for the most part are preventable. They aren't allergies, just negative responses to something you're introducing to your body, consciously or not. The Virgin Diet is a tool to wipe the slate clean, start from ground zero, detoxing the body naturally, and learning what foods are interfering with your system. It's the "right" place to start when looking to lose fat, gain energy, deter disease, and live a long and productively fantabulous happy life.

Were you aware that up to 20% of Americans show signs of battling with some degree of food intolerance? This is according to a study conducted by graduates at the *American Society for Nutrition.* The most common are to gluten, soy, and dairy. Showing symptoms mildly for the most part, which encourages this minor "annoyances" to be dismissed and never diagnosed.

To keep it simple, food intolerances often appear because the gut wall itself isn't as resilient as yesteryear. Particularly due to poor eating habits, alcohol and drug abuse, stress in general, medications, parasites and infections, and other environmental toxins that regularly circulate freely through your blood system. Over time, this will eventually take its toll in the form of disease. Food intolerance may be one of the first overt signals to take action in communicating this earning to you crystal clear.

Food sensitivities are often heightened with the exposure to all the unnatural chemicals and pollutants in our world. This increases the intolerances to additives and preservatives in processed foods - like Trans fats and MSG, and is linked to the hypersensitivities popping up left, right, and center towards food in general.

Specific Food Intolerances

Lactose, fructose, and glucose intolerances, are center stage when considering health and wellness and food sensitivities. Understanding their purpose, is going to help you make the connection between The Virgin Diet eating strategy, and food hypersensitivity. Making your new eating strategies that much easier to instigate and apply for life.

Lactose Intolerance

This is something that affects up to twenty percent of Caucasians, and an astounding sixty percent of the Asian and Mediterranean community.

Basic symptoms may include:

* Cramping and nausea
* Bloating and diarrhea
* Gas and vomiting

Lactose intolerance happens when there isn't enough lactase manufactured in your small intestine. Lactase is what breaks down lactose, so your body can use it. By age five, your body stopped making lactase, so most of us have at least some degree of intolerance here. If you have any sort of issues with your gastrointestinal tract, you might also experience symptoms of lactose intolerance.

The Virgin Diet will help you isolate your lactose intolerance, and learn how to better your overall health and wellness as a result. Experts agree, this "elimination diet" is an excellent tool in helping you figure out whether lactose intolerance is in your blood.

ACTION STEPS

- Use The Virgin Diet to eliminate foods that may be triggering tummy trouble, and slowly reintroduce these suspected trigger food, to determine exactly what milk-based foods are screwing up your system.

- Probiotics, slippery elm, zinc, and glutamine, are also options geared to help "fix" your gut, so you can tolerate milk products
- a trial and error process, but it doesn't hurt to try

Fructose Intolerance
In basic, fructose is a sugar in fruit, processed sugars, and table sugar. HFCS, is high fructose corn syrup found in many different processed foods to sweeten them. If your body isn't able to breakdown and absorb fructose, you're going to see the following symptoms:
* Bloating and diarrhea
* Gas and nausea
* Cramping and vomiting

Up to thirty percent of Americans are affected, and fructose intolerance is directly associated with IBS, or Irritable Bowel Syndrome. It's important you get tested if you have this disease, just to ensure you don't also have fructose intolerance.

ACTION STEPS
- The Virgin Diet will help you eliminate foods containing fructose, and direct you to slowly reintroduce them singularly, to see which ones work, and clash with your body.
- It's important to note many foods are sneaky here, and have fructose hidden within. Just like a pretty little Christmas package with a bomb in it. Foods like ketchup, barbecue sauce, and other pasta and meat sauces, have HFCS in them.

HF Foods to Steer Clear Of . . .
- Honeydew, mango, pear and watermelon
- Apples, coconut products, guava and tomato
- Star fruit, fruit juice, dried fruits
You are better off going with foods sweetened with glucose, including . . .
- Pineapple and rhubarb
- Citrus, grapefruits and oranges
- Grapes, various berries and kiwi

Chewing your food slowly and thoroughly, will also help with the digestion process. Stay privy to the fact overloading your system will only aggravate intolerances. So don't eat more Dreamy Triple Cheesy Cheddar Cheese Pizza, when you know just one bite sends you to the potty!

Gluten Intolerance

I'm sure you've heard of this one before. Gluten is a natural component found in rye, oats, wheat, barley, and spelt. It's used regularly in food production because it's favorable in the cost factor.

Gluten's Used Routinely in:

- Baked goods
- Meats and meat products
- Ice-cream and yogurts
- Cosmetics (not a food I know but still worth mentioning)

Symptoms of gluten intolerance may be . . .

* Gas, fatigue, bloating and cramping
* Nausea, anxiety, nausea and vomiting

ACTION STEPS

- Bet you guessed it! The Virgin Diet will help you eliminate all traces of gluten from your system, then isolate which foods work with your body, and which don't. You'll take all these foods off the menu, then slowly add them back one at a time. This is the only way to isolate if gluten intolerance is an issue for you.

- Whole grains are a good move here, and with all sorts of gluten-free products from which to choose, you can have your cake and eat it too for the most part if you venture carefully.
- Probiotics will help balance your intestinal tract, improve your gut quality, and decrease any inflammation within your intestinal tract.

29

Bottom line, is that food intolerance can sabotage your weight loss plans, and leave you frustrated and tubby. The idea is to figure out what foods interfere with the smooth running of your system as a whole, and replace them with nutritional choices that are easy on your digestive tract, and give your body all the nutrients it requires to zap free radicals, provide energy, get rid of fat, and make this all sustainable. It doesn't do you an iota of good, to work hard transforming your life habits healthy, to figure out days later you can't sustain these changes.

The Virgin Diet digs to the root of the problem and eliminates it. Food intolerances are exposed, giving you a solid base from which to build healthy eating habits, and a positive active and happy lifestyle for life.

My Thoughts . . .
Food intolerance and food allergy are similar but different. If you're allergic to a specific food, you really have no choice but to avoid it altogether. However, you can work with foods you may think you have an intolerance for. Some food intolerances come and go, and others are triggered by both internal and external factors. Often, such as the case with cheese in many instances, people can have some cheese, but too much will cause issues with their digestion. This is a trial and error process, subjective, and The Virgin Diet is a great route to discover where your body stands with all this.
Knowing the best foods for you is the first step in gaining control of your weight, health, and overall gynormous smile.

Benefits of Virgin Diet

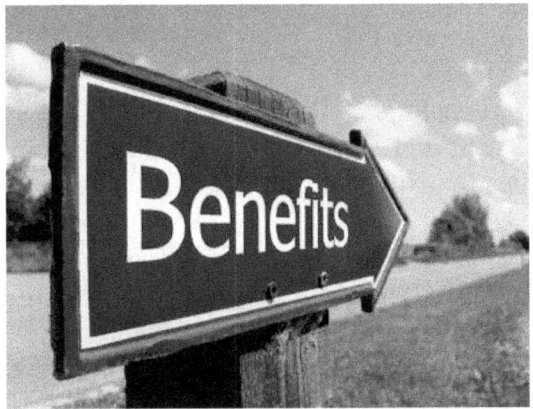

As with everything in life, there's crap and fantabulous. The Virgin Diet is one of those diets that sets you up for long-term weight loss success. With the added bonus of deterring disease, gaining energy, increasing your positive, and setting you up for a balanced and happy lifestyle, one that isn't going to change with the season, like most other diets.

Benefits are:

* *Lose Weight* - Certain highly reactive foods could very well be interfering with your natural ability to drop weight. The Virgin Diet addresses this, removing these foods, and slowly adding them back, to figure out which ones are tolerant with your body system, and which ones you best steer clear of.

* *Gain Weight* - Some people need to gain weight, and this diet enables you to get the right number of nutritional calories to do just that. Personalization is easy with The Virgin Diet, and you'll the peace of mind knowing you're gaining the weight you need the "healthy" way.

31

Sustain Weight - Most diets set you up to lose weight, then leave you out to dry. They don't have a plan to help you keep it off. Probably because the measures you took to drop fat were extreme to begin with. This diet re-programs your brain, while giving you the knowledge and "know-how" to make new healthy food choice habits, and incorporate enjoyable exercise into your every day. This is a lifestyle change that is easily sustainable if you choose that.

Reduced Inflammation - By taking the seven highly reactive foods out of your diet, you'll decrease inflammation, which is directly linked to just about every disease.

Improved Complexion - Removing the seven reactive foods from your body, will naturally improve your skin. It will regain elasticity, appear toned and smoother, have less breakouts, decreased dryness, and will appear younger.

Blood Sugar Levelling - When you're filling your system with simple sugars, triggering spikes in blood sugar levels, your mood and energy levels get walloped. Without a constant source of good food energy, you're stressing your system, increasing the chances of developing serious disease like diabetes, which is all about blood sugar levels.

Overloading Your System With Nutrients - On The Virgin Diet, you're loading your system with all sorts of vital nutrients, antioxidants, protein, calcium, and essential vitamins and minerals, that are going to build your body and mind strong, resistant to disease and illness, energy fatigue, and negative attitude about life in general.

Better Sex - This one deserves bold print don't you think? You are reading this correctly. Studies show this diet actually increases testosterone levels and libido. Makes sense, because if you're feeling great about your weight loss, sexy, and energized, why wouldn't you want to have great sex?

My Thoughts . . .
Most diets have more negatives than positives, particularly
those hugely popular fad diets. The Virgin Diet is a no non-
sense approach to figure out how your particular body reacts
to various foods, and it doesn't leave you hanging. This diet
works with you, to give you the knowledge of what your body
needs to gain energy, fight off disease, and help lose weight.

While making sure you have a diverse array of foods from
which to choose, that are going to make certain you feel good
about food physically and psychosomatically.

Eating is supposed to be simple and enjoyable. The Virgin Diet
shows you that's exactly how it can be. Supporting the ultimate
goal of keeping you slim and healthy for the rest of your life
without sacrifice.

Food Myths/Truths

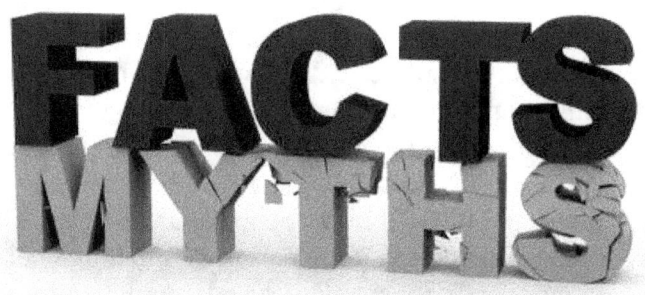

It's pretty tough to get away from the rumors that circling round, including the food myths that make us stress over fact or fiction. Here are a few mystic myths that may or may not be familiar to your ears. Regardless, it's time to debunk a few food mistruths.

Myth One - Never use a wooden cutting board for meat. This may sound like a food rule encased in stone, but surprisingly it's not true. Yes, bacteria gets down into a wooden cutting board when sliced with a knife. But research studies show this bacteria gets trapped down there, and doesn't make it back to the surface when properly cleaned. It dies in due time. Fact is, bacteria gets down inside the top layers of a plastic cutting board too, particularly if it isn't cleaned properly.

Bottom line is, you've GOTTA clean your cutting board properly after every use. Just base your buying decision on your personal preference, and don't make it about bacteria.

Myth Two - Dairy is the only route to sexy strong healthy bones.

This may have been what health experts believed back in the olden days, but times change, and with it the information on strong bones and dairy. Dairy does not mean just calcium. Dairy does contain calcium, but so does broccoli, leafy green vegetables, and tofu.

Dairy also has protein, and other essential vitamins and minerals. Try not to think absolutes with food groups because 99.9% of the time there are other options with a little digging.
Milk is also fortified with Vitamin D, along with numerous other milk products, essential for great health. Research shows that having long-term fantabulous bone health, means more than just Vitamin D and calcium. You need Vitamin K too, which is found in leafy green veggies and not in dairy products.

Magnesium also contributes to strong bones, which is found in oatmeal, potatoes and nuts and isn't in dairy items. Don't forget about building lean muscle, which helps support optimal bone growth. The list goes on forever and a day plus one.

Of course calcium is important in taking care of your bones, and calcium is found in dairy products. But this is no longer the end-all-be-all of strong bones. If you want optimal bones add plenty of leafy greens, and some nuts/oatmeal to your eating plan.

Not to stir the pot here, but experts question whether milk should even be drank by adults. Did you know that humans are the ONLY mammals that continue drinking milk after infancy. Well there is one other exception to the rules that I know of. My barn cats and dogs happily shared bowls of milk after when I was milking the cows, and filled up a few buckets with unpasteurized, body temperature warm milk. Like Christmas morning to them!

Myth Three - Eggs are going to send your cholesterol through the roof.
Saturated fats will trigger elevated cholesterol levels. Eggs do have small amounts of saturated fat but no Trans fat. But eggs are loaded with thirteen natural vitamins and minerals essential to good health. In other words, the trade off just isn't worth it. The benefits of eating eggs are just too awesome to pass up for most.

You might better use The Virgin Diet to eliminate other high-fat, high-calorie interference foods, that are standing between your weight loss and fabulous health.

Myth Four - You should always drink 8 glasses of water a day.
Talk about a "ho-hum" general rule. This myth was created when doctors were trying to convince the world to stay away from sugary drinks, and quench their thirst with crisp refreshing water instead. Yes, you should hydrate your body with water. It also helps cleanse your system, propelling it to function more optimally, and make you feel better, psychosomatically at least.

Just keep in mind the amount of liquid energy your body needs, is as unique as you are. The calculated amount your body needs depends on your metabolism, weight, height, body composition, lifestyle, health, and activity level to start. Factor overload if you ask me!

As a rule of thumb, most people need to look at their body weight in ounces, and cut it in half to figure out the water needed daily. Your body and mind needs water to function optimally, but this exact amount will vary daily. Some days you may need more, and others days less. It's best to start with 6-8 glasses each day, reflect on how your feel, see if this number makes sense considering your activity level, size, environment, and so forth, and adjust.

Myth Five - If you want to cook food faster, just add salt.
This is one of those myths that does ring true. Although the truth factor is so minute, you might as well ignore it. Experts agree, that salt does in fact alter the boiling point of water, but the effect is so small you'd have to dump a truckload in to make any real difference. Obviously this would make the water totally disgusting, so basically it's more accurate to say the salt changing the boiling point of water really isn't something you need to worry your pretty little head over.

Myth Six - Carbohydrates make you fat.
Bottom line is eating too many calories and not burning enough is what makes you fat. Eating too many high-calorie nutrition-less simple carbohydrates like white bread, pasta, pastries and sweets, inevitably makes you fat over time, along with increasing your risk of developing serious illness like cardiovascular disease, and adult onset diabetes.

Cold Hard Fact: There are huge advantages to getting the right about of complex carbohydrates into your system, including whole grain breads and cereals, whole wheat pasta, rice, and sweet potato.

Complex carbohydrates are loaded with fiber, and a whole whack of essential vitamins and minerals your body needs to gain optimal health. Moderation is the key, and never discount the importance of balanced eating, including healthy carbs.

Myth Seven - Beans and rice need to be eaten simultaneously or you aren't going to absorb the protein.
Proteins are combinations of amino acids - making everything from muscle to hormones. There are 20 amino acids in all, and your body only manufactures 11 of them. Meaning you need to get the other 9 from food sources. Animal sources offer up all 9 of the remaining amino acids your body needs, to absorb adequate amounts of complete protein. So meat sources are a great source of protein.

Experts no longer think you need to eat a specific combination of food, like rice and beans, at the same time to get the protein you need. What's more important, is that you take a time-out to look at your eating for the whole day. As long as you're getting these food combinations at some point during the day, it has just the same effect as eating them together at the same meal. *Awesome to know!*

Myth Eight - Searing meat seals in the juices.
This has been a debate for years. Some experts believe searing meat seals in the juicy, and you're going to get a moist and tasty meal every time. Truth is, you can seal in those tasty juices by searing your meat, but if you keep cooking it long enough at a scalding hot temperature, you're going to dry the crap out of it, rendering it juiceless.

The best advantage by searing meat, is that the Maillard Reaction occurs. That tasty browning process of the surface of the meat that's makes your mouth water. This in itself, makes the searing process worthwhile, juicy or not.

Myth Nine - Aluminum foil triggers Alzheimer's Disease.
For years experts thought aluminum levels were higher in Alzheimer's patients, than the normal populous. So, many healthy nuts just stopped using it completely. Moving forward with time, after years of studies, nothing scientifically conclusive and absolute surfaced to prove this claim, reversing the death sentence for aluminum foil.

In fact experts discovered, than any aluminum entering the system is absorbed by the kidneys and excreted naturally. Good news for everyone, particularly aluminum foil addicts like me!

Myth Ten - All calories are equal.
This is like saying to a hockey player, that all hockey sticks are the same. Are you freakin crazy?

Where your calories come from means *everything* in great health. It's your hormones that are signaled to react every time you fuel your body. And it's the *type* of food you eat, that tells these hormones their function.

If you eat a whole grain peanut butter and banana sandwich, your body is going to react differently, than if you eat a piece white bread with butter and a soda. The second option, is going to shoot your blood sugar levels through the roof pretty much instantaneously, and drop your energy levels in the bucket like your last paycheck. You're spiking your energy levels with sugar, and the consequence is short-term, leaving you hungry and without energy shortly after.

Just think how you felt a short time after your last candy bar. With the whole grain bread option, you aren't overloading your system with simple sugars. The complex carbs and protein you're giving your body will last longer, and instead of spiking your energy and blood sugar, you're providing constant energy longer. The fiber plays the part here.

This gives you what you need to build lean muscle, exercise longer, keep your energy levels up, and ultimately zap pesky fat. A definite plus in my books.

My Thoughts . . .
When I think about myths, I think of gossip. Mistruths that are set to cause hurt and turmoil. Getting to the bottom of these food myths, is going to give you the information you need to make better food decisions as a whole. The only way you're going to build an effective, efficient, and wholesomely healthy eating strategy for you, is to start with the cold hard facts. Use these food truths, to help create your solid healthy food plat-form from which to build.

Mental Factors to get Started

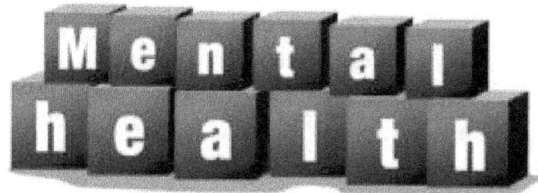

It doesn't matter what sort of changes you're set to make in your life, if your "mental" isn't on board, it just won't happen. When it comes to adjusting your eating, you're going to need all the advantages you can get, to make the right health changes for you. Smart moves that are going to set you up for LIFE HEALTH success.

Unfortunately for our society, the word "diet," is naturally re-flected upon negatively. An automated magnetic field of resistance is often present, before we even begin. Since your mind is ever-powerful, this makes it more difficult to view any sort of "diet" or "die" with a "t," in a positive light. Too bad the word meaning diet, wasn't "Christmas" or "party."

If you think or believe dieting is unpleasant or hard, it will be. In other words...

Your reality is what you make it.
By re-jigging your thinking on diet, and the like positively, you WILL make your new transition into healthier smoother and with less self-created resistance. If you can consciously remove the negative associating with an eating style change, and focus on all the benefits of it, you're going to succeed in making the changes, losing weight, and feeling fabulous, all in due time

FACT: According to the *Canadian Dietician Council,* it take up to SIX months of repeating an action to turn it habitual, and make it stick. This means you will go about your day not having to think about the healthy new behavior you committed to just six months prior. I'm sure fast learners get to this point a few months sooner. Point is, no matter what positive healthy eating, exercise or lifestyle change you're adopting, give it time to sink in so you don't have to think about it to do it. That just hurts your brain!

Your behavior here is either driven by your want to avoid pain, or the intrinsic need to feel pleasure. If you see dieting as gaining pleasure, you're going to increase your efforts naturally, gaining greater results as a whole. It won't be viewed as giving up or "killer work," but a labor of love. One you constantly make minor adjustments, in order to create your new and healthier "normal," when you eat.

So you can choose the scenic route or the direct one. Of you choose to look at dieting as all negative, or make it all about giving up all your favorite treats, you're consciously choosing to set yourself up to fail. A rumbling tummy, a whole whack of "not allowed," and constant tiredness, these thoughts will in time overcome your desire to take action to get blubber loss results.

However, if you can look to, and focus on the fantabulous benefits of losing weight, you're much more likely to succeed. Dropping pounds like flies will give you the energy to live YOUR life as YOU see fit. For many, the bonus of losing weight, enables you to enjoy slipping into your sexy pink and blue polka dot bikini, instead of hiding behind a XXX-large stinky black tent t-shirt come summer time!

Sad to report, one main reason people procrastinate starting a diet, or making any positive eating changes, is because they truly believe the cons won't outweigh the pros. The really believe there is too much sacrifice and too little gain.

FACT: *It really doesn't matter what anyone else thinks here but YOU!*
If you don't believe shrinking fact cells, dropping a few dress sizes, gaining energy, decreasing pesky aches and pains, deterring disease, and transforming toned and sexy, is a great load of moves for you, THEN IT WON'T. At least it won't stick for the long run.

Let's have a look at your conscious and subconscious mind.
Conscious Mind - It commands action
Subconscious Mind - It obeys
Your conscious mind . . .
* Recognizes data coming in
* Evaluates the situation
* Figures out what to do
* Creates goals and passes judgment
* Looks positively toward trying new things
* Thinks in abstract
* Holds short-term memories

* Has time measurement - past and present
* Ultimately programs the sub-conscious
Your Subconscious mind . . .

43

* Takes control of your unconscious bodily systems like breathing and heartbeat
* Triggers fight or flight response
* Dictates your emotional response
* Controls two automated learned responses
        - thinking or mental actions
        -physical actions like walking or running
* Holds memories
* Is programmed by the conscious mind
* Solves creatively
* Can't decipher harmful thoughts versus helpful
* Computes and stores incoming information in your memory
* Doesn't know real from imaginative

My Thoughts . . .
It's important to make sure your mental thinking straight, if you're going to attempt to change any of your engrained behaviors. Change is difficult, and your noggin controls success or failure. The mind is a powerful thing, driven by your desire, and external factors.

If you really do want to lose weight, gain control of your eating, and get healthy, it's got to start with positive thinking. It's all about mind over matter.

You are in charge of you, and your mental needs to understand The Virgin Diet is only going to help you in succeed in your master quest for good health.

Tips to Stay on Track (Third Cycle)

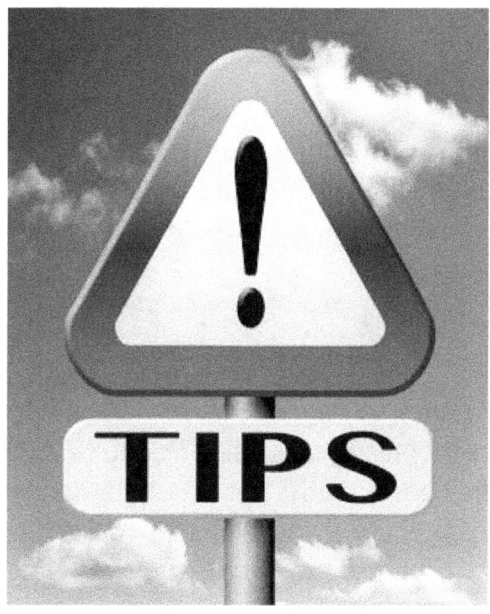

It's tough to stay on track when you're trying to transform healthy eating changes into habit. We seem to start off positive and strong, often losing our way just before reaching our "new" eating style.

The third cycle in The Virgin Diet Plan, is to create your eating plan for life. Using the foods that work for your body, respective of your likes and dislikes, what you prefer and what you don't like. It's not about right or wrong, but setting YOU up for success in permanent weight loss, good health, and wellbeing for life.

Here are a few thoughts that will help you stick to your plan:

45

* *Plan your meals in advance*. This will help you stick with what your body needs, not necessarily what you "think" you want.

* *Keep a diary of your thoughts and feelings to look back upon*. This helps inspire, keeping your focus forward toward at all the progress you've made.

* *Avoid sabotage triggers, particularly in the beginning steps*. If you have to stay away from going to the movies, or out for dinner for the first few weeks, then do it!

* *Take a picture of yourself and look at it anytime you're thinking of veering off course*.

* *Stick with all natural foods if you can*. Stay away from boxed and packaged foods, because they tend to be loaded with toxins that build up in your system over time, and interfere with fat loss, and good health. Just think about it for a minute. If you're eating chemicals and preservatives in processed foods that are foreign to your body, you can't possibly expect your body to know how to rid your body of them? Well it won't, forcing this toxin to find a tissue to hide in and lurk. This causes interferences with the regular smooth running of your system as a whole, affecting everything thing you do, think, and feel.

* *Make certain you don't have sweets and treats within arm's reach*. This means clear your house out of foods, that aren't supposed to go into your body. You're going to run into "weak moments, simply because you're human, and if you actually have to get out of your comfy chair, get dressed, and head to the market to cheat, you're less likely to do it. In other words, you're buying yourself some time to get your head on straight,

and make the best food choices for your weight loss, and great health.

* Try to dissuade your attention from television ads about unhealthy food, and magazine pages that are glorifying all the fatty unhealthy processed foods of the world. This little effort in removing temptation, will help you steer away from self-induced cravings. If your mind isn't thinking about your past eating habits constantly, that's only going to help you create a healthier present, and future.

* *Surround yourself with a positive support system that's going to help you stay a virgin.* You need people that are going to boost you up, and help you reach your goals. It's very important to be wary of those people looking to knowingly or unknowingly sabotage. People who you "think" want you to lose weight and get beautiful inside and out, but don't really want to.

Maybe your best friend feels really bad about her weight, or your boyfriend is starting to get insecure in himself, because you are starting to lose fat and look sexier to other guys? If so, they may "say' they're proud of your efforts and will support you. Truth is, they've be the first to offer you a big tub of popcorn at the movie theater, or tell you you're doing an awesome job, and deserve to be treated to a nice fattening dinner out, with a gynormous piece of chocolate cake.

I'm not suggesting you get paranoid, but it really is important you're careful who your supports are, in your quest to get skinny with The Virgin Diet concept.

* *Drink lots of water and don't get dehydrated.* You may not have to drink as much water as you think, but not getting enough can be dangerous. Water also helps you a little mentally when it comes to eating. Up front, water helps you feel full, and of course helps your internal systems run efficiently. By

creating the habit of drinking a glass of water before each meal, you'll decrease the likelihood of overeating. It's definitely worth a shot.

* *Using a small plate is a great strategy to make yourself think you are eating more.* This is another scenario of mind over matter, that's going to help you feel fabulous about adopting and using The Virgin Diet. Every little bit does help!

* *Rewarding yourself provides incentive and inspiration to keep on track with your diet.* This doesn't mean heading out for a tub of full fat ice cream, after you lose your first ten pounds. But it does mean treating yourself from time to time with things that make you truly happy. Maybe you are a shop-a-holic, and love shoes. Every month you may reward yourself with a new pair of shoes. Maybe you love reading, and will buy a new novel every week that you succeed in making your health better. It's up to you to figure out what's important to you, and make sure you utilize it to support positive growth centered on The Virgin Diet lifestyle.

VIP for You!
Foods Encouraged With Virgin Diet
* ***grain-fed beef, organic pork, farmed salmon, shrimp, lamb, free-range chicken and turkey***
* ***flaxseed, pea rice protein, hemp and chia seeds, almonds and walnuts***
* ***organic berries, kale, lettuce, tomatoes, asparagus, sweet potato, and avocado***
* ***brown rice , quinoa, oatmeal (gluten-free), lentils, and co-conut milk***
* ***xylitol, extra-virgin olive oil, and palm oil***

My Thoughts . . .
There are so many different strategies to help you stick with your new healthy eating plan. What's important here, is you

figure out what works for you, and make it happen. Always keep your eyes and ears open for new tips, to help you succeed in your transition to The Virgin Diet for life. New information is only going to fuel your determination, and renew your want/need/ and desire to succeed in weight loss, and all the positive health benefits attached.

Strategies That Make the Virgin Diet a Success Anywhere

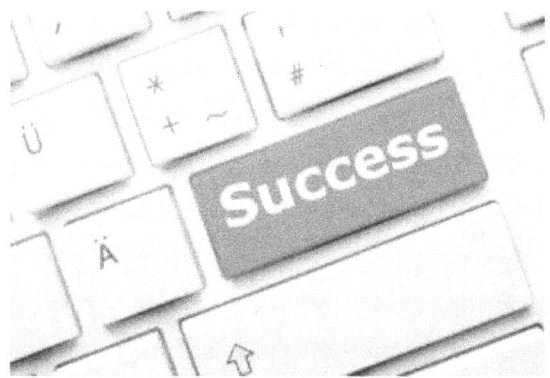

Eating right is tough, and when you're out and about, sometimes it's downright impossible. If you happen to be out of the country on business, the breakfast included with your stay may be advertised as healthy, but in reality consists of packaged muffins, white toast with butter, and bottled fruit juice. Hardly a high protein, good carb start to energize your morning!

When you are trying to lose weight, and make the "right" food choices, following a diet regimen often makes it that much harder. I also understand finding grass-fed meat, and tasty quinoa isn't that easy either.

If you've got food intolerances, this just makes eating outside your stomping grounds, more difficult. It's just too easy for a chef to add egg or milk, to thicken a soup or sauce. The Virgin Diet does have some steadfast rules, but it really won't take you long to become a natural in handling yourself outside of your home turf. Be patient and persistent, and you will prevail.

Here are some strategies to help you take positive action:

* **Be Adventurous** - Don't be afraid to mix and match on the menu. Maybe you are salivating over the broiled salmon, but don't want the mashed potato that comes with it, preferring the broiled spinach that comes with the chicken instead. Politely ask your server if you can please switch sides. Normally this isn't a problem. After all, you control the tip.

* **Ask to Clarify** - Please don't assume the chicken doesn't come with a milky cream sauce, or the sweet potato isn't deep fried. Just ask to be sure of what you are getting. Don't give yourself an excuse to eat the wrong things.

* **Start With Salad** - Studies show people who eat a small salad with a drizzle of olive oil dressing, tend to eat less calories overall. This just means, when you actually start to eat your meal, you aren't starving. Crazy hungry people tend to wolf down food, and not listen to their system screaming they're full.

* **Steer Clear of Gynormous Salads** - Salads aren't always your best option. Particularly if they have fried onions, bacon bits, croutons, candied fruit, and sweet nuts, and are served in a fancy fried taco shell. These are all items often accompanied with salads that aren't nutritional for you. Top one of these salads off with breaded fish or chicken, and full fat salad dressing, and you're better off having an order of fries and a cheeseburger - I kid you not!

If you want a salad with a whole mix of fresh veggies and fruit, and it happens to come with fried chicken and bacon bits, ask to make a change. Often skipping the bacon and cheese, and opting for grilled meat, and drizzling the salad dressing, will make this tasty salad nutritious for you too. This may take some time learning, but if you use your logic, ask questions, and follow your waistline, you WILL make the right foot choices for you.

* **How it's Cooked Matters** - Just because you are ordering chicken and veggies, doesn't mean it's healthy for you. Stay away from breaded, deep dried, sautéed in butter, crunchy, crispy, creamy, and glazed to start. These cooking methods often add loads of extra fat and calories to you dish that aren't necessary! Look for grilled, baked, broiled, poached, and barbecued instead.

* **Appetizers Be Gone!** - Except for basic salads with little or no dressing and clear soup, don't even allow appetizers on the table. This is just asking for trouble, particularly with that in-famous never-ending bread basket, garlic sticks, and cheesy mozzarella sticks to start. Most appetizers are just going to tan-talize your fat buds, and I'm telling you to leave them out of site.

* **3 Bite Rule** - If you are with someone that insists you try that triple chocolate devil cake, or have some creamy cherry cheesecake, you can. Just train yourself to take only 3 bites, then drop your fork, and ask the server to take the remains away. Make this habit, and you'll discover how much willpow-er you really have. Mind over matter does prevail, and you still get rewarded with some cake!

* **Don't be Afraid to Make Changes** - The menu is the "end-all-be-all." Substitutions are definitely doable in most cases, and all you have to do is ask. Maybe the restaurant has a fab-ulous low-fat meat dish, and you just don't want the creamy garlic pasta, but would prefer the steamed broccoli and as-

53

paragus. Just ask! Ask and you shall receive. That's how I work anyway.

* **Doggie Bag to Start** - It's a proven fact that restaurants serve meals 2-3 times the size your physical body needs. Ask for a doggie bag to start, and immediately stuff half of your meal into it before you even take one bite. This smarty pants move sets you up for success. This will help you deprogram your overeating, reminding your body and mind how to stop chomping BEFORE you're stuffed. This also sets you up for lunch the next day or maybe a treat for someone else.

Add Ons - Cause Long Term Healthy for Life is MORE than Just Smart Eating
Regular Exercise Like You Mean it!

Your body was built to move, and your mind function relies on regular exercise to get balanced. Intense exercise helps alleviate stress, induce energy, decrease annoying creaks and cracks, and help your physical internally and externally run more effectively.

Blowing through extra calories by interval training daily, lined up with your preferences and tolerances, will help you build your mental and physical stronger, increase metabolism, blast flubby rolls, increase motility, and enable you to enjoy a much happier and more productive life in all areas.

Muscle building is critical in maintaining strong bones, muscles, and supportive structure. It also burns calories at a higher rate than smaller celled, softer, and bigger fat. Intense cardiovascular exercise like biking, swimming, running, hiking, and power walking, help support strengthening heart and lungs to function strong with less effort, along with improving internal circulatory systems, providing healthy nutrients faster throughout your body though the blood stream.

I really could go on forever and a day here. The point I'm making is that regular intense exercise IS a part of a healthier, leaner, sexier you for life!

Sample Exercise -
*Cross-Fit Training
*Interval Circuit Training
*Biking and Resistance Exercises
*Weights and running or biking
*Swimming
*Hiking
*Weight Training and Intense Yoga
*Gardening With Effort

Social Balance
As humans, we're programmed to need routine social interaction in order to sustain good health. Research shows people that have regular social interaction life longer, perform better at work, weigh less, have more confidence, better jobs, make healthier food choices, and have a better overall outlook on life in general.

According to *WHO, World Health Organization*, social factors directly influence the health of an individual.

Smart Social Moves to Make -
*Make plans to get social with friends and family weekly
*Try new hobbies to meet new people
*Open your mind to romantic relationships, or work positively on the one you're in
*Talk regularly with a counsellor
*Ask for help when you need it
*Don't try and do "life" alone
*Learn to forgive and forget
*Seek out strong friendships
*Learn to open social doors, not close them

Hereditary
This factor directly affects your overall health and wellness, but it's not something to dwell on. It's not like you can change the fact that cancer runs in your family, or that your body was made with a teeny tiny upper portion, and is bottom heavy down below.

Focus on the positive your genetic makeup delivered, and take action against any negative health or lifestyle factors. If cancer runs prominent, make sure you get tested and work harder to make healthier eating, exercise, and lifestyle choices.

If you believe a "lazy" lifestyle is programmed in every one of your family members, make sure that's not the case with you by getting fit and healthy. Lead by positive action and maybe the rest of your family will eventually follow suit.

The bottom line here is, you need to take the information you can and reflect positively on it. Where you can make positive change you should, and where you can't just acknowledge it and forget about it.

Environmental Reality
Pollution and even negative lifestyle factors, chosen or not, will impact your good health. If you smoke, that's going to negatively steal your energy, turn your body ugly yellow, smother your oxygen stores, and slowly poison you from the inside out. This is a lifestyle/environmental factor you can change.

Living in a big city where pollution is an issue may be a little harder to escape, but it can be done. If your workplace sucks in the clean breathing department, you deserve to look for solutions that will make your working environment healthier for you.

The idea here is to look for both environmental and lifestyle factors you can improve on, and just get it done. Where there's a will there's a way champ!

My Thoughts . . .
It's important to make your dining out experiences enjoyable. For example, if you see something unhealthy on the menu, and know getting the fish broiled instead of fried makes the dish healthy, then muster up the courage to ask if you can have it prepared that way. More often than not, a restaurant is more than happy to accommodate. You don't have to sacrifice healthy eating when you're munching outside of your home. In fact, most fast food restaurants offer low-calorie, low-fat healthy alternatives for people that are eating to lose fat and get healthy. It even helps to do a little online research before picking your restaurant if possible. Knowing what you're going to order before you set foot in the restaurant, will deliver the peace of mind you can eat out, enjoy it, and still watch your fat pounds disappear.

Paradise in your brain.
When it comes to exercise, genetic makeup, social factors, environmental and lifestyle realities, it's up to you to do whatever it takes to make your life as a whole fantistico. NEWSFLASH! There is always going to be room for improvement, and it's up to you to engage the target and fire away!

Final Thoughts

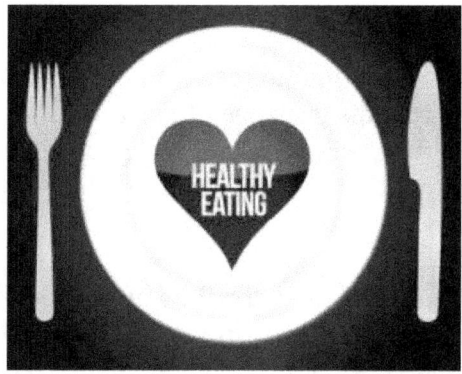

The Virgin Diet Supreme is a scientifically proven, logical strategy, supporting lifelong healthy eating habits that are fun, diverse, versatile, and exciting. You should be comfortable when eating, and blend in nicely in any social situation. This is exactly what The Virgin Diet Supreme encourages.

This diet makes sense, because it starts from the ground and gradually works its way up. In today's society, your body is susceptible to so many different interferences from the environment and genetics, to lifestyle and even medication based influences that you really need to keep an open mind to address a multitude of factors toward positive change.

Each of these unnatural scenarios may, or may not cause issue with the way your body absorbs and processes specific nutrients vital to your good health. As a beginning, by removing the seven foods people are most likely to react to, and re-introducing them slowly one by one, you're able to determine if these foods are causing trouble with your digestive process. If so, you can even determine whether or not your body can handle them in small amounts, or not at all. An example, is the common breakdown issues associated with milk and milk products.

Some people have a mild intolerance to milk, and may be okay with a glass, or perhaps one slice of pizza on occasion. Although anything more may cause bloating, upset tummy, and interference with the absorption of other important vitamins and minerals.

This diet helps you start with the food groups that YOUR body accepts best, and creates a diet that works for you. Helping you lose fat and build your body strong, energetic, and resistant to illness and disease.

I don't know about you, but that's all good in my books. Don't you think it's time to figure out the foods that suit you best, add to that better social, physical, mental, environmental, and lifestyle choices, and transform your health into fantabulous?

Last Thoughts…

*THANK-YOU for reading my masterpiece. I hope you learned a little something, or at least got a few smiles.
*I would appreciate a millisecond or three of your time for a quick review, to help me build my masterful book empire higher.
*Whatever you do, don't forget to smile, and of course, check out my website for more of my e-Book masterpieces: www.flawlesscreativewriting.com

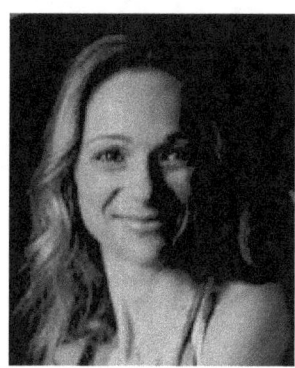

www.ingramcontent.com/pod-product-compliance
Lightning Source LLC
Chambersburg PA
CBHW070617290526
45790CB00002B/933